I KNOW
HOW HARD
YOU
WORK

Other books by Paul Sybert

The Dreamer and the Hummingbird	print/e-book	
Intimacy: My Journal	CD	spoken
Collection of My Poetry	CD	spoken
Across the Border	CD	music
Inspirational Songs	CD	music
Love Songs: Spread My Wings and Fly	CD	music

To contact Paul, e-mail: psybert@stny.rr.com

I KNOW HOW HARD YOU WORK

A Journey Through
Stroke Recovery

Paul Sybert

iUniverse, Inc.
New York Lincoln Shanghai

I KNOW HOW HARD YOU WORK
A Journey Through Stroke Recovery

iUniverse books may be ordered through booksellers or by contacting:

iUniverse
2021 Pine Lake Road, Suite 100
Lincoln, NE 68512
www.iuniverse.com
1-800-Authors (1-800-288-4677)

Because of the dynamic nature of the Internet, any Web addresses or links contained in this book may have changed since publication and may no longer be valid.

The views expressed in this work are solely those of the author and do not necessarily reflect the views of the publisher, and the publisher hereby disclaims any responsibility for them.

ISBN: 978-0-595-46079-3 (pbk)
ISBN: 978-0-595-69919-3 (cloth)
ISBN: 978-0-595-90378-8 (ebk)

Printed in the United States of America

I dedicate this book to my guardian angels. During my darkest hours as I recovered from a stroke, my guardian angels encouraged me constantly to overcome the obstacles I faced each day. They reminded me that God is good and would always do his part. They encouraged me to do my part and try. Each day I healed and got better. I thank God and my sweet guardian angels. They help me heal, they help me write, and they help me live each day.

A special thank-you to Debbie Winters, my editor.

Contents

Introduction

One day something happened to me. I was sitting at home in the living room, and I had a stroke. It was an ischemic stroke. The dictionary defines ischemia as a temporary lack of blood in an organ or tissue (the brain in this case). It was caused by a clot in my brain cutting off the flow of blood to the cells in my brain affecting the left side of my body.

The unthinkable had happened to me. I had a cerebrovascular accident, a CVA, or stroke. My arm and leg went numb, and I couldn't walk right. That's all I knew. I called 911 and was taken to the hospital. I had no idea that I was on a three-hour countdown that would affect the rest of my life. The important thing was that I received a drug that has to be administered in the first three hours after the stroke occurs.

That day, my life changed and became undefined, at least to me. At that point, life became "one moment at a time," every day. My job, I began to realize, was to redefine that life that had become undefined.

This book describes my healing experiences in my stroke recovery. I found that my daily practices, my affirmations, and my mental visualization, as well as prayer and meditation, were as instrumental in my healing as my physical therapy. That is the reason I have included them here. They are important to me, and I want to share them with you.

My first job is to recover from a devastating stroke. My second is to describe my recovery in such a way as to encourage those that have had a similar experience. It is intended to give you hope and to say "don't quit, don't give up, and look for new ways to love yourself along your own personal journey of recovery."

If you are recovering from a stroke or know someone who is, I hope this book helps you. This book is written in a workbook fashion. I have recorded my thoughts and feelings and have provided a space for you to do the same.

Chapter One:

The Ride to the Hospital

After the EMT squad took me out of my apartment on a chair, they put me into the ambulance and told me they would be using the lights and the siren. They told me so I would not be scared, I guess. But I wasn't scared yet, so it didn't bother me. It was hard to believe that I had had a stroke. Strokes happen to other people, not to me—or so I thought. Having a stroke seemed so far away until then.

It was still unreal to me—but I couldn't move my left side. At the hospital emergency room, the team did a CAT scan immediately. The emergency room doctor told me I had had a stroke, and it was a blockage stroke. They wanted to administer a drug called TPA, which is given to people with certain types of strokes to improve their recovery. It is a clot-buster drug that needs to be given within the first three hours after the stroke. It was dangerous, because it could have caused me to bleed to death someplace else in my body. The emergency room doctor said if it was him in my place he would take it. I told him, "Say no more, I'll take it. Do it, shoot it to me." But before they could give me the drug, my lower blood pressure number had to be 105 or less. After a few injections of medicine to lower my BP, I was a prime candidate for TPA. Just in time—it had been almost three hours.

Time was more important than I realized. By now I was scared, and appropriately so. I was in the sector of humanity that could have a stroke, and I did have a stroke—today—three hours ago!

"It couldn't happen to me," changed to, "It did happen to me." The emergency room team became angels working directly for the Almighty.

I had good care in the emergency room; but now I was acutely aware that this was serious, and I was in God's hands. Life as I knew it changed that day.

I didn't lose consciousness and had no headaches; my left side just went numb. I was in God's hands before the stroke, but I was aware of it now in a very real way. That day my life changed—and life became undefined, somehow.

Daily practices

Feelings: I am scared.

Goals: Get through the day.

What I'm grateful for: I am grateful for getting to the hospital quickly.

Progress: Not sure yet.

Reminder: I tell myself, "Whatever I need to do today, God will help me do it. I need also to remember that my efforts are incredibly important—and I need to hold in my mind the image of me completely well."

Mental exercise: I affirm, "The brain is a magnificent organ; whatever image of myself I hold in my brain, it will try to accomplish or make happen."

A place for you to reflect

My feelings:

My goals:

What I'm grateful for:

My progress:

Reminder:

Mental exercise:

Chapter Two:

The Next Forty-eight Hours

After the emergency room I was taken to an intensive care unit, where I could be watched closely for a couple of days. Since I had been given the TPA drug, I could still bleed out, so to speak. The critical time period for observation was forty-eight hours. Bleed-out could occur anywhere in my body, from ulcers I didn't know I had, or if I cut myself shaving, etc.

They put me in Gloria's unit. Actually it wasn't her personal unit, but she thought she was in charge, and everyone was afraid to tell her otherwise. Everyone was afraid of her but me. Don't get me wrong, I was leery of her. She was the type of nurse that you did not want to cross, but she was a good nurse and could help me a lot. We had a good rapport—at least, I thought so.

The hospital was full of Gloria stories. Many people would walk the other way to avoid a confrontation with her. Somehow, I couldn't resist this type of personality. I enjoyed matching wits and sparring a little.

We got on well for those two days in her unit as long as I remembered that it was her unit—a lesson the other hospital personnel had learned before I got there.

She shaved me before I left her domain. Either I was not to be trusted with sharp objects yet, or, if I was cut and started to bleed to death, she wanted to be the one to get the credit for saving me. I casually referred to Nurse Ratchet, but I really meant Gloria. Actually, before my time in hospitals was done, there would be many Nurse Ratchets—but that comes later.

When I got to "Gloria's unit," the hospital sent a speech therapist to see about my chewing and swallowing. The stroke had affected these areas, they thought, and they wanted to establish a diet that was right for me. Gloria told me that I should tuck my chin when swallowing, and it would be easier. I should also be careful with thin liquids because it was easier to swallow thick liquids than thin ones. Thin liquids made me choke at first. With thin liquids there was less time for the swallow/choke response to protect me. But I am stubborn and don't listen sometimes. Gloria had warned me. I hated it when she was right. She was always right. She said to chew the food on the right side of my mouth at first. Since the stroke had affected the left side of my body, it might be too easy to lose track of the food in the left side, and I might choke.

I mastered chewing and swallowing in a short time. The food was good. I was motivated; I was hungry. Amazingly, I didn't gain any weight during my thirty days in the hospital.

Before I left Gloria's unit I had a bowel movement. Nurses are very interested in bowel movements. On Gloria's watch, when a patient had to go, she brought in a portable potty. When she brought it into my room, she said, "Here!" and then called for two aides to put me on the special toilet. She also said, "Call when you are finished. And don't you dare wipe!" The process stripped me of what little dignity I had left. I thought my life as I knew it was over. I was wrong, but my life had definitely become undefined. I was now living in a new zone.

Daily practices

Feelings: I feel fortunate I received the TPA clot-buster drug.

Goals: My initial goal is to adjust to this new situation and get better.

What I'm grateful for: I am very grateful for prompt medical treatment.

Progress: Too soon to tell.

Reminder: I tell myself, "Whatever I need to do today, God will help me do it. I need also to remember that my efforts are incredibly important—and I need to hold in my mind the image of me completely well."

Mental exercise: I affirm, "The brain is a magnificent organ; whatever image of myself I hold in my brain, it will try to accomplish or make happen."

A place for you to reflect

My feelings:

My goals:

What I'm grateful for:

My progress:

Reminder:

Mental exercise:

Chapter Three:

Squeeze My Finger

When the forty-eight hours was up, and it was decided that I was not going to bleed to death, I was moved to the neurological unit. They held me in the neurological unit until a bed became available in the rehab unit of another hospital. They wanted to stabilize me medically. That means the neurologists wanted to get my blood pressure down and decide which medications to give me. They thinned my blood, lowered my BP, and reduced my cholesterol. They visited me periodically and examined me.

The exam amounted to two areas. They said, "Squeeze my fingers with your left hand and wiggle the toes on your left foot." They had me stumped with this exercise. If I could do those things, I wouldn't be in the hospital. So I worked very hard to squeeze their fingers with my left hand and wiggle the toes on my left foot.

After I had been in the hospital for a week, I was considered "stabilized" medically. I met the doctor in charge of the rehab unit at the next hospital, where I would be going soon. He didn't say very much. What he did say was blunt, and I considered him to be rude. At some point near the end of his short speech, he ducked around the curtain at the side of my bed, and I didn't realize it. Keep in mind that I could not see around the curtain at that point, and I didn't know where he was. I kept waiting for him to return, but he did not. Our first meeting left me with the feeling that I didn't like him very much, if at all—the doctor had a lousy bedside manner, blunt speech, and the nerve to leave my room without saying a word. Nevertheless, I was transferred to that hospital and his rehab unit a few days later.

My first impression of him didn't change very much, but the rehab unit had an excellent reputation. I was very happy to be there and knew that I would get the attention that I needed.

Daily practices:

Feelings: I feel well cared for on the neurological floor.

Goals: My goal is to sit up in the chair longer each day.

What I'm grateful for: Good medical care, good food, and kind nursing staff.

Progress: I sit in the chair longer and longer each day.

Reminder: I tell myself, "Whatever I need to do today, God will help me do it. I need also to remember that my efforts are incredibly important—and I need to hold in my mind the image of me completely well."

Mental exercise: I affirm, "The brain is a magnificent organ; whatever image of myself I hold in my brain, it will try to accomplish or make happen."

A place for you to reflect

My feelings:

My goals:

What I'm grateful for:

My progress:

Reminder:

Mental exercise:

Chapter Four:

On Your Feet

The marines have a saying that goes, "Off your ass and on your feet; out of the shade and into the heat." I worked for a marine for twenty-five years at one of my jobs. I got to know their ways by association. The rehab was a little bit like that, I thought. The tone was different on the rehab unit.

The food was good. They fed you well and worked you hard. Maybe it was like spring training camp. All I know is that I fell asleep after the physical therapy sessions at the end of the day. The therapists were tough, and there was not much sympathy—correction, there was no sympathy! But I liked it, and it was what I needed.

The therapists gave me my movement back, I guess you could say. For three weeks they pushed me into walking with my walker, using my left arm and hand to some extent. I was showering and bathing myself, dressing myself, and peeing standing up. I am getting a little ahead of myself; I did pee standing up right away, just not by myself. For days the nurses/aides insisted on being there. Their motto was, "You'll never walk alone, at least not on my shift. You'll never stand up alone either."

I could end the hospital part of this journey right here, I guess, if it weren't for the hospital procedures I was always trying to violate. Dependence versus independence was a topic that the nurses and the doctors were passive-aggressive about. Complete independence inside your room required an order from the doctor, and that was restricted to the day before you went home.

I fought with the doctor concerning many things, not just the independence thing. I waged my own private war with him about allowing me to have vitamins and natural remedies, like aloe. I lost almost every argument I had with him. What was I thinking? This was a hospital! Why did I think I could convince a doctor to use a natural-health remedy along with medicine? I fought the good fight, though!

In the rehab hospital I began answering my phone with, "Hello, Dr. Rehab's House of Pain." It made me feel good.

Daily practices

Feelings: I feel roughed up by the rehab staff. I feel angry, but at the same time I feel like I am in the right place to get better.

Goals: My goals are to adjust to the new situation and to do what I am told.

What I'm grateful for: Sitting up, using a wheelchair, learning to dress myself with help and doing minimal exercise.

Progress: I am doing life in a new way, with help from the rehab staff.

Reminder: I tell myself, "Whatever I need to do today, God will help me do it. I need also to remember that my efforts are incredibly important—and I need to hold in my mind the image of me completely well."

Mental exercise: I affirm, "The brain is a magnificent organ; whatever image of myself I hold in my brain, it will try to accomplish or make happen."

A place for you to reflect

My feelings:

My goals:

What I'm grateful for:

My progress:

Reminder:

Mental exercise:

Chapter Five:

Use It or Lose It

The idea behind rehabilitation after a stroke is to use the part or parts of the body affected by the stroke.

That is exactly what happens in rehab: the plan is to use it, use it, use it—and not to worry about how it looks. I was more than a little gimpy at first. I swore that I was trying out for the Special Olympics, but they kept pushing because …

Soon I would be going home. I was considered unique because I lived alone and had an independent lifestyle, and my home had some stairs. They knew that when they released me there would be no one at home to care for me, so they put me in the category of needing a little extra, I guess. They walked me longer and harder. They said, "You live alone, so we have to do this." They taught me to climb stairs. When they found that I was afraid of heights, they used a special stairwell, the one leading to the roof. They did their best to teach me to adjust, to be unafraid, and to move forward into the unknown into a life that had become "undefined."

They taught me to use a wheelchair, a walker, and a shower chair. We went through the routine of getting up from a toilet of regular height. The ones in the hospital were higher. We did a dry run with the shower chair. We talked about safety first—always, safety first.

I became a little sensitive to the fact that I had had arguments with most of the key players on the staff, and I didn't want to jeopardize my going home. So, for a day or two, I became unusually noncombative.

Daily practices

Feelings: I feel many feelings. I am happy for my progress, angry for being pushed hard, and scared when I try new things.

Goals: My goals are to adjust to the rehab unit and to learn all I can here.

What I'm grateful for: I am grateful for good food and good rehab and medical care. I am grateful to be learning skills that will eventually let me go home to live on my own.

Progress: I am progressing in many areas, mainly in gaining independence—dressing, exercising, and motivating myself—so I can leave the hospital.

Reminder: I tell myself, "Whatever I need to do today, God will help me do it. I need also to remember that my efforts are incredibly important—and I need to hold in my mind the image of me completely well."

Mental exercise: I affirm, "The brain is a magnificent organ; whatever image of myself I hold in my brain, it will try to accomplish or make happen."

A place for you to reflect

My feelings:

My goals:

What I'm grateful for:

My progress:

Reminder:

Mental exercise:

Chapter Six:

Preparing Me to Leave from the Start

I stayed in two hospitals. The first one, in which I stayed a week, was to treat me medically. The second hospital was a rehab facility. Different types of patients are taken there: stroke patients and people who have had operations. They are all given physical and occupational therapies and other therapies to help them be independent and use their bodies again. They are taught to walk with a walker and to use their arms and upper torsos, and they are given cognitive and speech therapy, if needed.

People who had had operations would eventually heal, use their arms and legs, and walk. The miracle was when this happened with people who had had strokes.

In the rehab unit, I dressed myself as far as I was allowed to. But I had to call for help when I wanted to stand up. It was hard to stand and pull up my pants at the same time.

Although it was hard for me to let people this close, at some point I started having a bit of fun with it. I would call for a nurse or an aide and say I needed someone to help me with the charming job of pulling up my pants—"Don't everybody rush right in here!"

This rehab wasn't for everyone, I was told. Some patients complained about the harshness and what at times seemed like callousness. But it is the fastest way to get better. It is a different kind of hospital; their methods are designed to produce results. I was helped physically, and I amazed even myself. But there was an emotional cost. They pissed me off most of the time. I saw through most of it, but some of the rules and a few of the people seemed arrogant without good reason. I found them aggravating. They sparked my ire and my adversarial nature.

I worked hard, and I was tired. It was an excruciating experience, but the angels were still there. Their light was probably even brighter because I was in a darker place.

I need to explain something that I haven't discussed yet. My body, or part of my body, did not work as it used to. My left side—arm, hand, leg, and foot—had changed or had abandoned me, or maybe a part of my brain had abandoned my left side. I had to invite my left side back to work with the rest of my body again. It sounds easy. But it took time and patience. I got very frustrated with myself. I made great progress with both my physical body parts and with patience for myself, but I still have a long way to go. This struggle is an internal conflict, as the really great conflicts are. Healing does happen; it takes time, and time does pass.

The harder I worked exercising the body parts, the more healing I got.

Daily practices

Feelings: I feel happy to be learning new skills to make me independent.

Goals: My goal is to learn all they can teach me in rehab.

What I'm grateful for: I am grateful for learning to get around better.

Progress: I am exercising more and using my wheelchair and walker better.

Reminder: I tell myself, "Whatever I need to do today, God will help me do it. I need also to remember that my efforts are incredibly important—and I need to hold in my mind the image of me completely well."

Mental exercise: I affirm, "The brain is a magnificent organ; whatever image of myself I hold in my brain, it will try to accomplish or make happen."

A place for you to reflect

My feelings:

My goals:

What I'm grateful for:

My progress:

Reminder:

Mental exercise:

Chapter Seven:

Outnumbered but Not Discouraged

One of the things I realized from the beginning in the rehab hospital was that I was outnumbered, and most of the staff stuck together. I wanted to take my vitamins, and the doctor would say vitamins were bad for me, and the nurses would nod *yes*. They eventually agreed to give me two vitamin Cs and one vitamin E. I was very grateful. But when I asked about beta-carotene, a vitamin and food supplement that is beneficial in the body's absorption of necessary nutrients and is also an anticarcinogen (cancer preventive), the head doctor said, "What's that?" I knew that I was in for a struggle. It's a good thing I didn't ask if I could have selenium. It would have caused quite a stir in the hospital, and I could have been in for the fight of my life.

I was given to understand that the good doctor didn't believe in vitamins. I was under his care. He would not authorize any more vitamins. I realized I was in his house, and I had to play by his rules. So I took my Vitamin C and E and was happy.

I knew I was outnumbered, but I didn't feel whipped. I mean, I was getting what I needed: good food, vitamins C and E, the right medications, and physical therapy to teach me to use my left hand and left leg. I was learning to function with my left side. But I couldn't leave it there. Knowing I would not win in a direct argument with the good doctor and his staff, I took my fight to another level. I argued with the doctor every chance I got.

After a while, realizing there were more of them and only one of me, I relaxed and went along for the ride.

My sense of humor kicked in, or I should say my warped sense of humor kicked in. My ally in this hospital's bureaucratic madness was Chuck. Chuck tested me on a regular basis to determine the damage and the areas affected by the stroke. He seemed okay to me, maybe because I liked his sense of humor. Anyway, he was my confidant and confessor. When the day wasn't going well, and when I had another argument with the staff, I talked with Chuck.

Daily practices

Feelings: I feel angry many times in the rehab unit. I am very confrontational with the rehab staff. I feel as if they gang up on me to make me do it their way.

Goals: My goal is still to learn all that the rehab unit can teach me.

What I'm grateful for: I am grateful to be learning new skills and slowly getting better.

Progress: My progress is slow. I can do new things, but I have to depend on other people.

Reminder: I tell myself, "Whatever I need to do today, God will help me do it. I need also to remember that my efforts are incredibly important—and I need to hold in my mind the image of me completely well."

Mental exercise: I affirm, "The brain is a magnificent organ; whatever image of myself I hold in my brain, it will try to accomplish or make happen."

A place for you to reflect

My feelings:

My goals:

What I'm grateful for:

My progress:

Reminder:

Mental exercise:

Chapter Eight:

Tested and Retested

As I mentioned, Chuck was the "tester." He knew where the stroke was located in the brain. His job was to determine which areas of the brain and my behavior were affected. I read stories, and he asked me questions about those stories. He timed my answers. He turned the radio on to distract me as I was tested. He did this day after day. I told him I was never good at these tests.

I almost flunked the third grade because of my lack of reading skills. I confessed that I had picked a career path of mostly math at the beginning in college so I wouldn't have to read much. I got my degree in electrical engineering. I was both awed and thrilled with how much math was involved. There was some reading also. I did what I had to, but that didn't mean I liked it.

I assured him that I had had most of the deficiencies he tested me for prior to the stroke. He tested me anyway. I told him I thought the women therapists were very pretty. I tried very hard not to provide details, like some of them had "nice asses." He assured me that was wise. He said the psych ward was just one floor up, so I'd better exercise some verbal restraint.

I no longer felt that *gimp* was a bad word. Though one of my therapists cringed a bit when I used it, I no longer felt either good or bad when I saw a physically challenged person. I had a kind of affection for "gimps." Now, I was one.

Daily practices

Feelings: I feel that rehab is a foreign place for me. I have to work hard to stay within their boundaries and limits.

Goals: My goal is to do what it takes to leave rehab and go home.

What I'm grateful for: I am grateful to learn new skills to make me more independent.

Progress: I am improving. The progress is very slow.

Reminder: I tell myself, "Whatever I need to do today, God will help me do it. I need also to remember that my efforts are incredibly important—and I need to hold in my mind the image of me completely well."

Mental exercise: I affirm, "The brain is a magnificent organ; whatever image of myself I hold in my brain, it will try to accomplish or make happen."

A place for you to reflect

My feelings:

My goals:

What I'm grateful for:

My progress:

Reminder:

Mental exercise:

Chapter Nine:

If It's Not Broke, Fix It Anyway

One thing you have to be careful of in the hospital is that they may try to fix something that isn't the main reason you're there. It sounds good initially, but it may not be.

When the nurse measured my urine, she told me that after I had peed there was still urine in my bladder. She did an ultrasound; there were 130 cc of urine still in my bladder. She said I might need a medication called Flowmax, which helps people pee more. She told me, "You are just under the cutoff point. If you had retained 150 cc I would have had to give you a catheter." That was a rude awakening. They had already done just about everything else, so I was happy that they didn't put a tube up my penis and install a catheter. It was scary, though. I didn't want to enter the hospital for a stroke and leave with a tube in my penis, or even spend the rest of my time there with a catheter. I decided that Flowmax sounded like the better of two evils.

I started to think that maybe I should just keep my mouth shut, but then I thought, *no, I just need to pick my fights a little better*. I was starting to adjust a little. I was grateful they didn't get me with that catheter thing, but it was too close for comfort.

Daily practices

Feelings: I feel I have to do what they say. I don't like it. I feel angry.

Goals: My goal is to go home.

What I'm grateful for: I am grateful for good food.

Progress: My progress is too slow for me—but fast enough to get me out of here!

Reminder: I tell myself, "Whatever I need to do today, God will help me do it. I need also to remember that my efforts are incredibly important—and I need to hold in my mind the image of me completely well."

Mental exercise: I affirm, "The brain is a magnificent organ; whatever image of myself I hold in my brain, it will try to accomplish or make happen."

A place for you to reflect

My feelings:

My goals:

What I'm grateful for:

My progress:

Reminder:

Mental exercise:

Chapter Ten:

The Fun Stuff

One of my therapists was a pretty young woman of maybe twenty-five. I called her "the princess." She constantly told me that I said inappropriate things. I was careful, but not careful enough for "the princess." One day while I was in therapy, sitting on a long workout bench, she sat down beside me—right on my hand. She turned bright red and moved over. Now the thing is, my left hand was palm down. We had just been working on exercises with the forearm and flipping the wrist. I asked her if this was a test to see how fast I could flip my wrist. I told her that I was doing well with my rehabilitation and getting better, but that I wasn't that good just yet. I wasn't quite fast enough. It did make me work harder to recover, though. There was no way I could just let moments like those go by unnoticed. A sense of humor kept me going.

When old guys like me have strokes, the hospital staffs up with women therapists who are young and pretty. It's so we have something to live for, I guess. After a particularly hard workout, I heard a pretty woman therapist say, "Is there anything we can do for you?" I said, "A lap dance would be nice!" Shame on me!

The Princess would constantly say that I was so inappropriate. I think she wanted to send me to the fifth floor (the psych ward) after my time in rehab was over. Therefore, I stayed safely on my side of the line. Part of the humor is knowing where the line is. As my rehab time neared its end, I became a little more careful, for fear I would not be released.

They came at me with their procedures and rules and regulations, and I used humor to stay afloat as best I could. It was definitely one against the many—I was the one and they were the many!

Daily practices

Feelings: I feel like having some fun in this restrictive environment.
The rehab staff purposefully screws with me, so I give it back as best I can.

Goals: My goal is to have fun. I have my limits. Within those limits I enjoy myself immensely.

What I'm grateful for: I am grateful for the good food.

Progress: There are times I feel as if I am standing still, but I am making progress, I know.

Reminder: I tell myself, "Whatever I need to do today, God will help me do it. I need also to remember that my efforts are incredibly important—and I need to hold in my mind the image of me completely well."

Mental exercise: I affirm, "The brain is a magnificent organ; whatever image of myself I hold in my brain, it will try to accomplish or make happen."

A place for you to reflect

My feelings:

My goals:

What I'm grateful for:

My progress:

Reminder:

Mental exercise:

Chapter Eleven:

Regular Coffee

Other than vitamins, my biggest fight while I was in the hospital may have been that the hospital cafeteria would not give me regular coffee. I was used to regular coffee. I wanted regular coffee.

Most of the time, in both hospitals, I struggled with this issue or procedure. What you have to understand is that in the patient database I was given a heart diet—low sodium, low cholesterol, low fat, no caffeine. I was okay with low sodium, low cholesterol, and low fat. But I wanted my coffee with caffeine. I had to fight the system from day one on this. I spoke with the dietitian, the doctors and nurses, and, finally, I was allowed to have regular coffee. It was put on my diet. Thank God—no more sneaking around and conning nurses for a cup of regular coffee. Now, let me say that the food in both hospitals was excellent. I loved the food. I was easy to please, I guess. I had been cooking for myself for several years. I had nothing to compare the hospital with, so, to me, it was great. Now the diet was complete. I could legally have regular coffee.

Daily practices

Feelings: I am feeling frustrated, and I am determined to work within the system to get what I need.

Goals: I want to learn all I can and go home—and meanwhile, get my coffee.

What I'm grateful for: I am grateful for regular coffee.

Progress: I feel like I am making progress, by being heard by the hospital system, when I am allowed to have coffee. This is a boost for my morale. It makes me feel good physically and mentally.

Reminder: I tell myself, "Whatever I need to do today, God will help me do it. I need also to remember that my efforts are incredibly important—and I need to hold in my mind the image of me completely well."

Mental exercise: I affirm, "The brain is a magnificent organ; whatever image of myself I hold in my brain, it will try to accomplish or make happen."

A place for you to reflect

My feelings:

My goals:

What I'm grateful for:

My progress:

Reminder:

Mental exercise:

Chapter Twelve:

Not Under My Care,
You Don't

Along with the fight for vitamins, which surprised me, I had an even bigger battle trying to get permission to have my own aloe drink. Aloe drink is refined from the medicinal aloe plant. Native Americans have long called it the burn plant, because of its healing qualities on burns, cuts, scrapes, and bug bites. Since it has been refined for internal use, it has been utilized for many other healing properties. I have found that it helps reduce my back pain. I have taken aloe for years, and, no, it didn't cause the stroke. The fight to take a capful of my own aloe with my juice in the morning was harder than I thought. I asked a friend to bring it to me in the hospital. When I didn't get it, I realized that it had been confiscated by the nurse. The doctor would not okay it. The nurse researched aloe on the Internet, and after a lengthy discussion, it was decided I couldn't have it. I asked the doctor point blank, "Why?"

He said he didn't know what it was. I said, "Why should I suffer because you don't know what it is?" He said, "You are under my care, and while you are under my care I won't authorize it for you." So, no aloe for Paul.

Now, compare the following story, with the aloe story. Hmmm …

One evening I was experiencing difficulty swallowing. I told the nurse. She called the doctor, and he prescribed a medication, which I took that evening, and I went to sleep. The next morning when I awoke my speech was slurred. I was disturbed by my slurred speech. I was told by the doctor and the nurses that the medication had a five-day half-life, meaning the slurred speech would go away in five days. I didn't believe it. So I asked for another CAT scan to see if there was any change in the stroke.

Finally they relented and gave me another CAT scan. A neurologist visited me too, I am guessing, to allay my fears of the stroke widening. They all said that my slurred speech was due to the medication and would most likely be gone in five days. After five days I still talked with a slur; when I asked the doctor about it, he said to just give it time. At the end of my stay, I asked him again, "Was it the medication, or did the stroke move?" He said the stroke probably moved. The "movement of an ischemic stroke" is a term doctors use to describe the movement of a clot in the brain that affects another part of the body. He said he thought so all along. I asked why the last CAT scan didn't show the stroke moving to affect my voice. I was told that sometimes the CAT scan doesn't show the movement of the stroke.

The bottom line is that doctors give out drugs easier than vitamins or aloe or regular coffee! I say this with tongue in cheek, to some extent.

I struggled with the doctor. I struggled with the nurses, but the nurses only carried out what the doctor said. I was told that nurses are the doctor's handmaidens. I thought that was well said.

Daily practices

Feelings: I feel angry. I won the coffee fight and lost the aloe fight. I also feel devious.

Goals: I am determined to get the aloe, so I took the battle underground.

What I'm grateful for: I am grateful I could at least get the nurse to put the aloe in my nightstand so I can have it when she is not looking.

Progress: I put the aloe in my juice in the morning when the nurse leaves the room.

Reminder: I tell myself, "Whatever I need to do today, God will help me do it. I need also to remember that my efforts are incredibly important—and I need to hold in my mind the image of me completely well."

Mental exercise: I affirm, "The brain is a magnificent organ; whatever image of myself I hold in my brain, it will try to accomplish or make happen."

A place for you to reflect

My feelings:

My goals:

What I'm grateful for:

My progress:

Reminder:

Mental exercise:

Chapter Thirteen:

The Last Roommate

I was more than a little fortunate with roommates. I prayed every time I got a new one. I am sure they did too.

Leo was my last roommate while I stayed in the hospital. It is hard to sum up a person like Leo, a natural storyteller, in just one chapter. When he spoke, you could hear an accent that sounded like Boston. Born in 1923, he was from New Hampshire. But he went to college at Northeastern in Boston, where he played football.

I spent most of the time with Leo telling him he should be writing the stories he told. I don't know whether he will or not.

The first thing I noticed about Leo was his magnificent command of the English language. What stands out in my heart is the spiritual light that he brought into my life at a very dark hour. He is Catholic, and although I am not, I quietly took part each time Leo received Holy Communion. Each day he did his morning prayers. He did his, and I did mine. He loved his family and revered his wife. He had nicknames for his children and grandchildren. Leo was scheduled to go home the day after I was.

Shortly after Leo arrived, my voice had altered somewhat. They told me the stroke may have moved. I had to work harder to talk and enunciate each word. I have a good voice, and this bothered me a lot. The day my voice was affected, I talked very deliberately. When I spoke to the therapist, I noticed that I sounded so deliberate that I almost sounded like someone else. That day I sounded like John Houseman in the movie *Paper Chase*, but later I guess it was more like Jack Nicholson. Now my voice is more like my own. I have practiced a lot, though.

Just because I talked funny didn't mean that I quit talking. Talking was too important to me.

When Leo began to tell his stories I listened, and I began to take notes. I'm not sure why, really, but he was an awesome storyteller. My taking notes was an automatic response, I guess. His stories made "good copy." Many of them involved sports, about which I knew very little. But during the time that he was my roommate, his light filled my darkness.

Daily practices

Feelings: I really like Leo; he is a good man. I am lucky to have him as a roommate.

Goals: I want to learn all I can and go home.

What I'm grateful for: I am grateful for getting better slowly.

Progress: I am making progress, but it is so slow.

Reminder: I tell myself, "Whatever I need to do today, God will help me do it. I need also to remember that my efforts are incredibly important—and I need to hold in my mind the image of me completely well."

Mental exercise: I affirm, "The brain is a magnificent organ; whatever image of myself I hold in my brain, it will try to accomplish or make happen."

A place for you to reflect

My feelings:

My goals:

What I'm grateful for:

My progress:

Reminder:

Mental exercise:

Chapter Fourteen:

Angels in the Hospital

Angels are of two varieties: seen and unseen. I know there are the unseen angels. I am convinced they helped patients like me sleep better at night. They gave us courage and the will to struggle against the odds and the circumstances we found ourselves in. The unseen angels brought the right people into the field of medicine.

Now I want to focus on the seen angels: the kind people, the compassionate people, and the ones with big hearts. Any institution of higher learning can train the mind, but the angel part of the person is on the inside: the heart, the kindness, the soul. God trains this part over a lifetime.

When a person's life is interrupted and it becomes undefined for a time, that person may question himself or herself. Some patients are in the position of needing some extra help from angels. I want to recall some of the angels that touched me in some way. Most of them were just doing their jobs and were good at it. Maybe it was their words, a look in their eyes, or something extra they did that was more than what was required. Maybe it was just some part of them that made them who they were. But what they did had a positive effect on me. God used that positive effect to encourage me at what seemed to me to be a dark time.

Daily practices

Feelings: I feel grateful for the angels in the hospital, both seen and unseen.

Goals: My goal is to heal.

What I'm grateful for: I am grateful for the healing I have experienced so far.

Progress: I use my wheelchair and can move it down the hall with my feet. I can walk to the shower at night with my walker. The nurse walks beside me. The only way the staff will let me shower is if I walk there.

Reminder: I tell myself, "Whatever I need to do today, God will help me do it. I need also to remember that my efforts are incredibly important—and I need to hold in my mind the image of me completely well."

Mental exercise: I affirm, "The brain is a magnificent organ; whatever image of myself I hold in my brain, it will try to accomplish or make happen."

A place for you to reflect

My feelings:

My goals:

What I'm grateful for:

My progress:

Reminder:

Mental exercise:

Chapter Fifteen:

Angels I Met Face to Face

What I recall are first names. All I want to recall is first names.

Mary

Mary was a nurse practitioner at the intensive care unit in which I stayed right after being transferred from the emergency room. She was pretty, with black, curly hair. She had an infectious laugh. At a time when I was low emotionally, I heard her laugh in the evenings. Each time I heard her laugh, I smiled. I asked if she would come to see me. When she came into my room I saw just how pretty she was: the dark hair, pretty brown eyes, and a beautiful smile. She shook my hand. Her hand was coarse, not smooth, and I knew there was a part of her life that some didn't know about and couldn't see on the surface. I asked what other work she did. She said she lived on a farm. In her presence I felt a depth about her that was as enchanting as her good looks.

When I saw Mary it was the evening shift, and the lighting in the hospital was lower than during the day. Her skin appeared to be a beautiful shade of bronze or brown. She looked like a princess to me.

She would be gorgeous in any light. She was either the most beautiful woman I had ever seen or God was telling me that this life was wonderful and not to give up just yet. I think I had begun to wonder if I still wanted to be here. Bottom line: her laugh cheered me up more than once.

Ryan

Ryan was the male nurse in the emergency room when I was brought to the hospital. As soon as he got my blood pressure stabilized with an injected drug, he started giving me TPA. TPA is a clot-buster that dissolves the clot that causes the stroke. This frees up the brain cells around the dead cells to do what the dead cells did before the stroke. This clearing away the clot in the brain assists greatly in the recovery.

Ryan was reassuring in his own way, with his presence. He had a certain believability about him that was comforting. When I was transferred from the emergency room to the intensive care unit, I didn't expect to see him again. His job as an emergency room nurse was done. But two days later, when I was moved to the neurological unit, he came to see me when his shift was over. Somehow, this stood out to me. This was above and beyond the call of duty. The nurses on that unit knew him; he had worked there before the ER.

Kyla

Kyla was the nurse on the night shift on the neurological unit. She was young and very skilled and had a nice manner. I liked her. She was consistent, acting the same each night. I felt that she always had time for me, and I appreciated that. She knew Ryan and had worked with him. Both she and Ryan were going to school, studying to become nurse practitioners. She was cute. Again, God wanted me here for now.

Shelly

Shelly was a nurse's aide on the evening shift and was very kind. I felt a good connection with her and gave her all the chocolate gifts I had received for the nurses. She was good with the other patients too; I could tell.

She was complimentary and supportive. She was the nurses' favorite, and I could see why. They thought of her as their daughter. She brought out the flirt in me.

Kimberly

Kimberly was on the day shift. She cleaned my room, and I enjoyed looking at her. She was a pretty chocolate woman who I lusted after in my mind. She cleaned my room two times one day, so I was treated twice. I watched every gorgeous move she made twice that day. She had pretty brown skin and black, curly hair. There must have been a lot of really sick guys in that unit. There was a high concentration of really pretty women.

Wendy

Wendy was the nurse on the evening shift on the neurological unit. She was very personable. She was gentle. She was likable. She made the evening seem more homey, somehow. So you ask, "Was she pretty?" Yes, she was. Was she young? Not really. She was younger than me. What stood out were her kind eyes. She had such kind eyes that if she hadn't been married already, I would want her, whatever her age.

This was a good unit for me. I stepped into something really good in this hospital—everything but the stroke; that wasn't good.

Debbie

We went back a long time. She came to see me as soon as I was admitted, and a few other times, too. I was flattered that she even remembered me.

I knew Debbie ten years ago. When she visited she looked exactly the same as she did ten years ago. I know the years showed on me, but they did not show on her.

She was encouraging about the stroke and the rehab I would be going to. Her son worked there. He said, "Mom, they work miracles there." I like miracles, so in my mind I started getting ready for one.

I think God was getting my attention with all these angels, which more than offset the disconnected, undefined event in my life that brought me here. My outlook is that there is no miracle, no good thing, that is beyond God.

So I am getting ready for my miracle. The angels and pretty women are added blessings.

Chuck

Chuck was the speech pathologist in the rehab hospital. He tested me to make sure that my cognitive skills had not been affected by the stroke. He would give me stories to read and ask me to answer questions about them. "We want to make sure that your attention span wasn't affected by the stroke," Chuck would say. He was a good person to talk with to lessen my discomfort and frustration.

He had a good sense of humor. I was told he was tricky, but I found him to be like me and enjoyable to talk with.

Alice

Alice was a nurse's aide. She was my midnight angel. She rotated and worked on any shift. She was one of the few that didn't have an agenda. She was just good to me. She was my friend, and I appreciated that.

One night, there she was in my room. It was midnight. I said, "Is that you, Alice?" Alice said, "Yes it's me." She then smiled that big Alice smile. She made my night (or day) special. All I knew was that it was good to see a friend.

Alice was pure. She was fun. The others were so focused on hospital procedures. I fought with people, but the fights were about procedures. Alice wasn't that way. We had some good conversations, and I enjoyed her company. Had she not been there I would have missed her. She was very real to me—still is. I wonder if she thinks about me today. I think so. I hope so. She was my midnight angel.

Daily practices

Feelings: I love these angels. They give me hope.

Goals: My goal is to heal.

What I'm grateful for: I am grateful for the angels I meet here. They help me realize how real God is to me in the healing process.

Progress: The real-people angels lift my spirit and encourage me mentally to get better and heal physically (so I can leave the hospital!).

Reminder: I tell myself, "Whatever I need to do today, God will help me do it. I need also to remember that my efforts are incredibly important—and I need to hold in my mind the image of me completely well."

Mental exercise: I affirm, "The brain is a magnificent organ; whatever image of myself I hold in my brain, it will try to accomplish or make happen."

A place for you to reflect

My feelings:

My goals:

What I'm grateful for:

My progress:

Reminder:

Mental exercise:

Chapter Sixteen:

Home at Last!

I am sure the hospital staff was as glad to get rid of me as I was to be leaving them.

I asked a friend to take me home from the hospital. As I entered my apartment with my walker, I saw the place where I lived very differently now. It was still the place that I called "home," but what I saw now was a series of obstacles. The first challenge was the staircase that greeted me as soon as I entered the front door. I had learned to go up and down stairs in rehab, including stairs much scarier than these. But this set of stairs was in my apartment, and I had to navigate them as I had been taught in the hospital. I am proud to say that my first challenge was a success.

It has been a month now since I've been home. I'm doing well, I think. I feel something subtle. I touch my left hand with my right hand. My right hand feels everything, but my left hand feels partially. I understand it with my head. But my left hand feels prickly, as if it is still half-asleep. It is waking up slowly. The unusual part is that the feeling is returning slowly enough that I don't know how it will be in another three months or so. I never know how the story will end, only that it will get better.

There is something else I need to remember. Everything is different now; it has been redefined. It gets better each week, but it is not the same as before the stroke. My thoughts in the beginning were that it would all come back: functionality, feeling—everything I had before would come back the same. The truth is that it is coming back, but different. I am sure that is hard to believe if you haven't experienced it. But that is the way it feels to me.

There is something else I need to explain. Before the stroke I enjoyed my solitude and spent a lot of time alone. When I was taken to the hospital, I had people around me constantly. In the hospital I associated having people around me with getting better. When I first got home I felt that I needed people around me so that I could get better. After a few weeks I realized that wasn't the case. My recovery doesn't depend on having people around. It is about what I do on a daily basis, like taking care of myself and exercising. It depends on my believing that I will get better and on seeing it happen. It relies on my doing hard things, like using the stiff hand gripper with my left hand. I struggle with it but keep using it, and my hand begins to get better.

As time goes by I find that I really do enjoy spending time alone, and I am still getting better. My progress is a function of me and not of the other people. It is also a function of time.

At home, my recovery truly depends on me and my efforts. It also depends on my vision of me getting better. God gives me what I am envisioning. He is meeting me in the place of my expectations. If I expect to get better, I do get better.

The hard part for me is having patience with myself. Healing from a stroke is a slow process—at least it seems slow to me.

Daily practices

Feelings: I feel happy to be home and alone.

Goals: My goal is to heal.

What I'm grateful for: I'm grateful to be alone.

Progress: I feel my progress will be greater here at home.

Reminder: I tell myself, "Whatever I need to do today, God will help me do it. I need also to remember that my efforts are incredibly important—and I need to hold in my mind the image of me completely well."

Mental exercise: I affirm, "The brain is a magnificent organ; whatever image of myself I hold in my brain, it will try to accomplish or make happen."

A place for you to reflect

My feelings:

My goals:

What I'm grateful for:

My progress:

Reminder:

Mental exercise:

Chapter Seventeen:

Exercise and Courage

Today I reached a new milestone. My first thought was to write it down and share it with you. After my shower I stood up to dry off with my towel. I stood up with no support from my AFO, or ankle-foot orthotic. The AFO is a bracelike device made for my leg to prevent my ankle from turning and spraining under my own weight when I walk. Now, that's progress! There have been other moments of progress that I am proud to report as well. Keep in mind that I now measure progress differently, in smaller ways than I used to. You may also.

About three weeks ago, while walking around my apartment, I noticed that I carried my walker as much as or more than I used it! I folded it up and put it aside. From that point on I walked on my own. My style was wobbly, but I was walking.

Last week I went out for a haircut. I needed gas for my car, though. After filling the tank, I thought, *I've come this far; why don't I visit my favorite restaurant?* So I did—another milestone, another bit of progress. I had removed the limitations on myself. I was on a roll that day. After dinner I was ready to go home.

Two days later I had an appointment to have blood work done. While I was in the neighborhood, I had the car's oil and filter changed at the local garage. On the way home, I stopped to get a few things at the drugstore. I was tired at the end of this day—tired but proud of myself.

About a month ago, before going to bed, I started doing several half-deep-knee bends, with the focus on the left leg. I put my hands on the bed, removed the ankle-foot orthotic, and did the exercises. At first it felt awkward and very weak. Over time it is getting stronger, I think.

I have been doing exercises for my upper body and for my lower body since I got home from the hospital. About five weeks ago I added hand exercises with my squeezers, using my left and right hands. It is difficult to do the exercises with my left hand, but I am making progress. I can now touch my left thumb to the top digit of all the fingers on my left hand. I couldn't do that in the beginning.

A few weeks ago I ordered an exercise bike and had it put together. It sits in my living room in front of the TV. Its unique position reminds me to use it daily. I am doing twenty minutes a day this month, and the plan is to progress one minute a day each month until I reach thirty minutes a day.

This week it will be three months since I had the stroke. I was told in the hospital that the three- to six-month time frame is an important time for functionality to return.

I am working hard. I believe that functionality can return at any time. It happens gradually, with exercise and hard work. I have to push myself—and it is very important that I do push myself.

A friend does reflexology on my feet and sees me every other week. I tell her what I am doing, and she sees my progress and says that I am courageous—and maybe I am. I am doing what I do to get the strength and functionality back. When I walk now without my walker, I walk from point A to point B, just as I live one day at a time. I don't look at the long distances, just point A to point B.

I don't know whether I am being courageous or whether I just want my independence back. I love my freedom and independence like never before. I don't want to be dependent on someone else. I am not afraid to ask for help, but I love depending on me. I also depend on God like never before.

God is a great healer, and he has endowed human beings with great ability to heal. I am aware of it like never before. I remember the adage "work like you are doing it, and believe like he is doing it." I live by this affirmation now.

I talk about my affected foot and leg, and walking. At this point in my recovery, I had to lift my left foot purposely when I walked, so I didn't catch my foot or toe on the rug. I worked on these motor-control issues a lot because that was a huge challenge for my stroke-affected side. I used both hands to eat, to type on my PC, and for other sensitive jobs. Turning pages in a book was fun. It had to be fun. I had to refrain from belittling and berating myself for using my left hand for close work. I used my humor as much as my hand, I believe.

When I think of motor control and using my left hand, many times I need to tell myself the joke about the gimp eating ice cream. Using the affected hand to hold the ice-cream cone, I struggle to bring it to my mouth. It winds up in the middle of my forehead. Remember, this is a joke. I usually get much closer to my mouth—but you get the idea. There is more to life than ice-cream cones. I typed this book on my laptop and used access codes and passwords. Maybe I will play the guitar again as I sing the songs I have written. Or maybe life will take me on a new and different adventure. I will still hold onto the vision of my getting better each day. This image, this vision, will take me where I need to go. It will help me do what I need to do.

Daily practices

Feelings: I feel more independent on my own at home, and I like it.

Goals: My goals are to do all I can do safely, and to heal.

What I'm grateful for: I am grateful for my independence and my solitude.

Progress: My progress is small each day.

Reminder: I tell myself, "Whatever I need to do today, God will help me do it. I need also to remember that my efforts are incredibly important—and I need to hold in my mind the image of me completely well."

Mental exercise: I affirm, "The brain is a magnificent organ; whatever image of myself I hold in my brain, it will try to accomplish or make happen."

A place for you to reflect

My feelings:

My goals:

What I'm grateful for:

My progress:

Reminder:

Mental exercise:

Chapter Eighteen:

My Tears Come
Flowing Out

Before, when I was inspired or touched emotionally, I felt that I could control it somehow. Now, when I feel touched emotionally and near tears, I just cry. The tears roll out, and I cry. My voice is full of the crying, and I no longer have the same control I used to have. The control may return with time, but for now it is gone. Maybe it is a form of grieving a loss. Maybe the tears fall whenever they have a chance. The feelings may be there just below the surface, awaiting their turn to be experienced. I don't know if this will change with time. But for now it is this way.

Music is more intense because of this, especially when I hear certain types of music. Particularly, folk music and acoustic music bring the feelings to the surface. Looking at my guitar, which I used to play with both hands, is acutely emotional. I don't know whether I will ever again use my left hand the way I used to, playing the guitar. Playing the notes and chords requires a high degree of manual dexterity.

I think at times that my life is taking a turn. I feel that the stroke may be a kind of bend in the road for me. I may not write music anymore. I may just write prose. My life is being redefined, as I've said, and my writing is being redefined along with it. My life is evolving and changing. It was doing that before, but it is different now because the change is stronger.

Daily practices

Feelings: I feel sad and cry while I watch acoustic music being played on TV—maybe because I feel I may never play it again with my left hand.

Goals: I work hard with my physical therapy. One of my goals is to improve my left hand's manual dexterity.

What I'm grateful for: I love my independence and my solitude.

Progress: I make small amounts of progress each day, sometimes maybe too small for me to see.

Reminder: I tell myself, "Whatever I need to do today, God will help me do it. I need also to remember that my efforts are incredibly important—and I need to hold in my mind the image of me completely well."

Mental exercise: I affirm, "The brain is a magnificent organ; whatever image of myself I hold in my brain, it will try to accomplish or make happen."

A place for you to reflect

My feelings:

My goals:

What I'm grateful for:

My progress:

Reminder:

Mental exercise:

Chapter Nineteen:

Adjustments Needed

Ankle-foot orthotic. In the rehab hospital an ankle-foot orthotic was made for me. The stroke had rendered my left ankle weak and unable to support my weight. I needed the ankle-foot orthotic, AFO, to walk. I still do. I can walk without my walker, but I am dependent to a great extent on wearing my AFO. That may change with time; I don't know.

I ride my exercise bike and hope that my left leg and ankle will grow stronger. I hope that they will strengthen to the point where I won't need my AFO to walk. I may always need it; right now, I do.

The shower chair. When I shower I use a shower chair. I remove my clothes and my shoes and my AFO, and I sit on the shower chair. The shower chair stays in the bathtub. I need it when I shower, because it is difficult to stand up without wearing my AFO.

I wonder if my ankle will grow strong enough so that I don't need my AFO, and then I won't need to use a shower chair. Maybe with time; I don't know. The shower chair is doable. It just makes traveling a bit trickier.

The changes are doable. I can adjust to the redefinition of my life. I have my independence. I can live my life as I did before the stroke, to a large extent. I am grateful for that. I lived alone before, and I can now. I depend on other people for certain things. But I can adjust. Each day I do adjust my life and my lifestyle.

Daily practices

Feelings: I feel frustrated sometimes, because I have to adjust to my new life with obstacles to deal with and to overcome.

Goals: My goal is to do what I have to do each day and know I am getting better.

What I'm grateful for: I am grateful for all I can do. I am grateful I am healing.

Progress: My progress is in small amounts, too small to see. I can see my progress over longer periods of time, like a week or two or even a month.

Reminder: I tell myself, "Whatever I need to do today, God will help me do it. I need also to remember that my efforts are incredibly important—and I need to hold in my mind the image of me completely well."

Mental exercise: I affirm, "The brain is a magnificent organ; whatever image of myself I hold in my brain, it will try to accomplish or make happen."

A place for you to reflect

My feelings:

My goals:

What I'm grateful for:

My progress:

Reminder:

Mental exercise:

Chapter Twenty:

Taking Stock
of My Progress

It is easy to live each day and not notice how much progress I have made. There are days when I try something new, and it becomes routine. It represents progress, and I want to continue doing it. I admit that I push the limits a bit. I push myself and do things that may be considered risky. But in my heart I feel ready, like the day I folded up my walker and began walking without it.

A baby doesn't count the number of times he falls. He is driven by a spirit of adventure as he tries new things. Other people watching him may be holding their breaths and thinking what he does is risky or dangerous. The bottom line is that I am beginning again, like the baby. I am older than he is, but I have to be willing to experience setbacks and have bad days as I progress. There are definitely good days. Soon it will be five months since the stroke. I have pushed myself and have made great progress.

Lately I have been doing some walking at home without my ankle-foot orthotic. I remove it now when I ride my exercise bike. The exercise without the orthotic helps to strengthen my left leg. My muscles and tendons, my ankle, and my knee are improving. I still use the orthotic for walks outside, for strenuous activities, and as a general rule. But I spend more and more time with it off.

Today I visited the rehab hospital and the therapists and nurses who helped me after the stroke. I showed off how much I have progressed. I enjoyed their reaction and surprise. I saw happiness in their eyes for me. They are good-hearted. I saw a side of them that I knew was there—a full-blown kindness and happiness that I am doing so well. I visited with many of them and finished my visit by having lunch in the cafeteria.

Something that is different about me now is the way I look at people who are physically challenged. I see them through new eyes. Before, I would have seen their handicap; now I see something else. I see what they do, how hard they try; I see their sense of humor. I see more inside them. I identify with them. There is a similarity to me, and that is what I see. I see us as equals. I am sure I saw them before, but it is different now. Now, "I am that too."

Today at the hospital I saw Chuck. We had some time to talk. He said the brain is always developing new neural pathways, which are the connections between brain cells. New neural pathways develop around the old dead cells to continue brain function. I hope I am quoting him correctly. But the gist is that the brain always provides the person with progress. Even five years later, studies have shown, with therapy there is progress. The brain never quits trying to provide us with progress as it works with the body after a stroke.

One of the therapists asked me if I was playing my guitar yet. I said not yet. But the point is that I don't know how much I will progress. I don't know how much will come back. My brain is doing a new thing. It is adjusting and developing new pathways for the neurons to help my body work better. God is doing a new thing in me, as the Bible says. I was told that the period between three and six months is a time of great return of function. Now I believe that progress continues for as long as you believe that it does. I have learned to not quit and to always have hope. My sense of humor keeps me moving forward. It keeps me afloat.

I don't want to finish this book too quickly. I want to capture on paper a sizable portion of my recovery. I am convinced a human being can do whatever he or she can envision. My intention is to share my recovery experiences with you. It is important to know that I am not alone in my struggle. Part of me wants to write this book slowly because I am always getting better. And I don't know how good I will get. I am beginning to think that the progress I make is ongoing. I feel it is a journey and not a destination.

It is a good day today. I have pushed myself, and I am tired. I feel good.

Daily practices

Feelings: I feel frustrated for many reasons. I am too close to my progress to know what it is.

Goals: My goals are to heal and to be more patient with myself.

What I'm grateful for: I am grateful for my progress. I know I am progressing. I am grateful for all God helps me with. I can see his gentleness at work in my life.

Progress: I am progressing each day; I know I am. Sometimes the progress is more obvious. It makes me want to try even harder. I push myself. I push myself too hard some days, and I find where my limit is for that day. It is okay. I try to always push the limits of the stroke recovery.

Reminder: I tell myself, "Whatever I need to do today, God will help me do it. I need also to remember that my efforts are incredibly important—and I need to hold in my mind the image of me completely well."

Mental exercise: I affirm, "The brain is a magnificent organ; whatever image of myself I hold in my brain, it will try to accomplish or make happen."

A place for you to reflect

My feelings:

My goals:

What I'm grateful for:

My progress:

Reminder:

Mental exercise:

Chapter Twenty-One:

The Imaginary Line

When a stroke affects one side of the body, there is an area in the middle that I have begun to call the area of "shared services." Draw an imaginary line down the middle of the body dividing the left and the right side. In the middle zone there are the eyes, the throat, the chest, the stomach, the intestines, and the elimination functions. My point is that after a stroke these areas are trying very hard to get back to normal, whatever normal is. I need to remember that these functions may be adjusting as well as the rest of me is adjusting.

Crying, swallowing, choking, digestion, and elimination functions are all adjusting. This is just my theory, but I am sticking to it for now. Therefore my advice to myself is, "Be patient with yourself."

The stroke affected my left side, but if something is wacky in the middle, I have to be patient with those areas too.

It is simple, really. When I drink liquids or eat food, I have to be more careful of choking. When my body says to go to the bathroom, I head in that direction. I listen to my body. When I cry now, it is not as controlled as it used to be.

Your tears are very special. They are your dreams talking to you. They will help you navigate to where you need to be to accomplish what is yours to do. They are part of your guidance system. I may not be able to play the guitar anymore, but I still need to write and create.

My goals may shift and change direction, but I still need to honor them in my life. My tears will lead me to my dreams and to the goals of what I need to do.

Daily practices

Feelings: I am happy to be making progress, however small.

Goals: My goals are to heal more quickly and to be more patient.

What I'm grateful for: I am grateful for all that does not need healing.

Progress: My progress is slow, but I am becoming content with that.

Reminder: I tell myself, "Whatever I need to do today, God will help me do it. I need also to remember that my efforts are incredibly important—and I need to hold in my mind the image of me completely well."

Mental exercise: I affirm, "The brain is a magnificent organ; whatever image of myself I hold in my brain, it will try to accomplish or make happen."

A place for you to reflect

My feelings:

My goals:

What I'm grateful for:

My progress:

Reminder:

Mental exercise:

Chapter Twenty-Two:

Give the Therapists
Their Due

I complained about the physical therapists while I was in the hospital, but the truth is that they showed me how to get better. They were God's instruments to get me out of the hole the stroke had put me in. "He lifted me up also out of a horrible pit … and set my feet upon a rock." (Psalms 40:2) I complained that the physical therapists were gruff, but the truth is that I needed that push to get better.

When I came home I did everything they showed me. I continued on my own. I focused on the weakened side of my body to make it stronger. I pushed myself and exercised. I pushed my limits hard. I tried to do it safely, but I did it. My voice had been affected by the stroke. That happened while I was in the hospital. So I used my voice and talked on the phone. I worked hard to sound like my old self. At first I pronounced each word very clearly and distinctly. My goal was to sound like me again. Work, work, work; talk, talk, talk; exercise, exercise, exercise—that's what I did. Sounds boring maybe, but I did what the therapist taught me.

Since I live alone, I play the role of both patient and therapist in my recovery. I push myself, and I hold a vision in my mind of myself as a healthy and creative and productive person. My vision of myself is very important, I think. I see me getting better and healthier every day. That is what I tell myself. That is what I believe that God is helping me do.

Daily practices

Feelings: I am happy to be doing my own physical therapy.

Goals: My goal is to get better each day.

What I'm grateful for: I am grateful for my solitude and my healing. Thank you, God.

Progress: I am making slow progress.

Reminder: I tell myself, "Whatever I need to do today, God will help me do it. I need also to remember that my efforts are incredibly important—and I need to hold in my mind the image of me completely well."

Mental exercise: I affirm, "The brain is a magnificent organ; whatever image of myself I hold in my brain, it will try to accomplish or make happen."

A place for you to reflect

My feelings:

My goals:

What I'm grateful for:

My progress:

Reminder:

Mental exercise:

Chapter Twenty-Three:

Maintain Your Vision
of Yourself

I work daily on the vision of myself that I hold in my mind. I see myself as getting better. Day by day I exercise and work hard to get back my functionality. Each day when I trip or do gimpy things that cause me to be impatient with myself, I renew my patience with myself. Each day I form and re-form an image of myself healing and recovering. My image, my vision of myself, has to become the new yardstick with which I measure myself. My vision of myself is what I use for my goal—not the clumsy things I do each day, but what I see myself becoming in my mind. My image of me, my vision of me, is my goal. It has to be that way for me to succeed with this new adventure. And it is an adventure.

Since day one of the stroke, each day has been an adventure. I have to use humor to lighten the moments that become too serious or too harsh. I push myself hard. But I also have to keep humor close at hand. I use the affected side for as much as I can. So, you can imagine what life each day is like. I walk. I stub my toe on my left foot and say unbecoming things about myself and the wall and whatever else you can imagine.

The bottom line is for me to hold tightly to the vision of myself as getting better each day. No matter what I manage to do on any given day, I focus on my vision of myself getting better. It is sometimes tiring to do this. So when I get tired, I take a nap. I don't have to remind myself to take a nap; I just take one.

Daily practices

Feelings: I am happy to know that my vision of myself is very important to my success and healing.

Goals: My goal is to do what I know is healing me.

What I'm grateful for: I am grateful for my health.

Progress: My progress is slow but sure.

Reminder: I tell myself, "Whatever I need to do today, God will help me do it. I need also to remember that my efforts are incredibly important—and I need to hold in my mind the image of me completely well."

Mental exercise: I affirm, "The brain is a magnificent organ; whatever image of myself I hold in my brain, it will try to accomplish or make happen."

A place for you to reflect

My feelings:

My goals:

What I'm grateful for:

My progress:

Reminder:

Mental exercise:

Chapter Twenty-Four:

Beware of the New Attitude

Having a stroke is a life-changing event. It is a serious, near-death experience. When this realization sinks in, something happens with your thinking. It did with me.

Time is a precious resource. I began to think of all that I wanted to do, to accomplish, and of who and what were important to me. I wanted to give the people and things that I love their rightful place in my world. And I wanted to tell them that I loved them. Something else happened as time went by: I began to feel less limited. In the beginning, right after the stroke, I felt incredibly limited—and then the feeling of being limited fell away. I still had to address things that related to my stroke, but in my thinking I began to entertain new ideas: things to do, to accomplish, and to let myself think about. I can't explain it, really, other than to say that time is short on this earth, and I wanted to do what was mine to do. I began to focus on goals and accomplishments, and I began to set out to get things done, like writing this book. The limitations fell away, and I thought about doing what I wanted to do.

Before, I may have thought, *I can't afford to do that,* and now I think, *I can't afford not to do that.* I want to take a train trip on the "American Orient Express" and visit our national parks on the journey from Salt Lake City, Utah, to Albuquerque, New Mexico. I want to visit Tuscany, in Italy. I want to publish this book. There are many things that I now want to do. So, I say to myself, "Beware of when the limited thinking goes away. You never know what will happen next." There is a feeling of joyous anticipation that sets in. It fills the body and the mind. When I awake in the morning, I never know exactly what I will do by the end of the day, or where I will go, or what I will get myself into. Beware of unlimited thinking. It may take you places you never dreamed of. God is a good God. So, between the two realizations, watch out!

Life becomes an adventure. Buckle up.

Daily practices

Feelings: I feel that anything is possible for me to do. God is helping me do things.

Goals: My goal is to heal and get completely well.

What I'm grateful for: I am grateful for my eyesight and my hearing and my ability to speak. I have so much.

Progress: My progress is enhanced by realizing what I already have.

Reminder: I tell myself, "Whatever I need to do today, God will help me do it. I need also to remember that my efforts are incredibly important—and I need to hold in my mind the image of me completely well."

Mental exercise: I affirm, "The brain is a magnificent organ; whatever image of myself I hold in my brain, it will try to accomplish or make happen."

A place for you to reflect

My feelings:

My goals:

What I'm grateful for:

My progress:

Reminder:

Mental exercise:

Chapter Twenty-Five:

Progress Is Ongoing

It has been nearly two years since the stroke, and my progress is ongoing. I find that my healing is still dependent on the same three main ingredients: my belief that God is good and helps me daily; my own daily essential efforts, exercises, and physical therapy; and my vision of myself getting better. It is so important for me to hold an image of my healed, well self in my mind. In this chapter I want to outline the exercises and therapy that I do each day. I also want to mention my view of my progress.

Daily exercise program

1. Meditate, pray, and read my daily books.

2. I exercise with hand squeezers, using both hands, to improve manual dexterity. I do several repetitions. The set I use is for weight lifters and is very stiff for me. I use the same set as I did before the stroke. My theory is that if is hard, it is good for me.

3. I lift ten-pound hand weights, one in each hand, and do several different curls and presses (for my arms and shoulders). While holding the hand weights, I do several half-deep-knee bends, then go up on my toes several times.

4. I do floor exercises for a ten-minute period, morning and evening. While lying on my stomach and arching my back, I flutter kick both legs, keeping knees straight. I do warm-up exercises first, which include push-ups from the knees.

5. I ride an exercise bike for thirty minutes at a level-three difficulty. It is very boring but helps to strengthen my legs, knees, glutes, lower back, and even ankles. This may be the hardest exercise I do.

6. Before going to bed I do more half-deep-knee bends, leg stretches, and exercises going up on the toes. Sometimes I try to see how long I can stay on my toes. I try hard to tire my legs so I sleep better.

Progress (as I see it)

1. I can walk with a cane and no other support.

2. I no longer use my ankle-foot orthotic. Not using it strengthens my entire leg, knee, and ankle.

3. After many months of riding my exercise bike, my thighs have strengthened to a point that I can stand up from a sitting position with just the use of my legs. I don't need to push off with my hands. I do sometimes, but I don't need to.

4. I ask for help from other people when I need it, as when I bring groceries down into my basement apartment from the car in the garage upstairs.

5. I am as loving and patient with myself as I can be.

6. Sometimes I go out to eat, both for the food and to flirt with the waitress.

7. I continue to write and do what I love. I live a simple life and enjoy as much of it as I can.

8. I don't put goals or plans out of my reach. If I really want to do something, I find a way. Life is too short to say "I can't."

9. I do have limitations and accept them as best I can.

10. I still dream and consider my dreams to be one of the most important parts of my life.

Daily practices

Feelings: I feel good about my healing and my life.

Goals: My goals are to heal and to enjoy my life each day.

What I'm grateful for: I am grateful that I can write this book.

Progress: My progress is slow. God's help is sure.

Reminder: I tell myself, "Whatever I need to do today, God will help me do it. I need also to remember that my efforts are incredibly important—and I need to hold in my mind the image of me completely well."

Mental exercise: I affirm, "The brain is a magnificent organ; whatever image of myself I hold in my brain, it will try to accomplish or make happen."

A place for you to reflect

My feelings:

My goals:

What I'm grateful for:

My progress:

Reminder:

Mental exercise:

Chapter Twenty-Six:

Merchant of Hope

I remember waking up in the hospital, the first night after the stroke, with a very anxious feeling. The reality of the stroke was beginning to sink in. At first I denied it had happened. I knew I could not move my left arm or leg—or anything on my left side. From that moment of acceptance on, I began to focus on what I could do: what I could control, what I could change, what I could do. My right side worked fine. Lying there in bed on my back, I realized I could also turn onto my right side by grabbing the side rail on the right side of the bed with my right arm. I had a choice: sleep on my back or on my right side. I felt better knowing I could do something. Then I went back to sleep.

There is an old saying, "You can't change or control anything beyond your nose." You can't change or control anyone but yourself. With the stroke, however, there were times that I couldn't even control myself. That was frustrating and discouraging. At first my left arm and leg would shake at times. There was a lack of control on my left side. As time progressed, control returned to my left side.

One day while my left arm was shaking, I said with my thoughts and in my mind, "Stop that," and I noticed that it stopped. It sounds simple, but it was the beginning of a new effectiveness in my stroke recovery.

I would use my mind to help my body. I would also hold a vision of my well self in my mind. That image in my mind became a goal that my body would automatically work toward.

Over time I have regained control on my left side. I can now do many new things with my left arm and hand, and my left leg and foot. The boring exercises are paying off slowly; they are returning control of my left side to me.

One day I was in a restaurant by myself when I realized one of my shoes had come untied! I said to myself, "Oh crap, my shoe is untied." A man at the next table overheard me and offered to tie my shoe. (His wife, sitting with him, appeared to be a stroke victim also.) I was touched by his kindness and willingness to help, but I thanked him and said I needed the practice. That man and that incident lifted my spirits, and I felt more connected with the world, somehow. I felt less alone. I was touched by the kindness of a stranger. He knew how hard his wife worked at her recovery, and I am sure he knew how hard I worked at mine.

There were times when I wanted someone to know how hard I worked, how hard I tried. If you are reading this book and you have had a stroke, I know how hard you try. I know how hard you work at your recovery, and I love you for it. I know how important it is for you to know that someone knows. I am proud of you. If people want to classify this book as little more than a "cheerleader's cheer" for those who have had a stroke, that's okay! My main desire is to give you hope. I am less an author and more a merchant of hope.

Daily practices

Feelings: I feel hopeful, and I try to spread that hope to other people who need it.

Goals: My goal is to heal completely.

What I'm grateful for: I am grateful for all of me that does not need healing. I am grateful for my eyesight, for my hearing, and for my ability to speak, to think and reason, and to remember.

Progress: I have made great progress. I can tie my shoes.

Reminder: I tell myself, "Whatever I need to do today, God will help me do it. I need also to remember that my efforts are incredibly important—and I need to hold in my mind the image of me completely well."

Mental exercise: I affirm, "The brain is a magnificent organ; whatever image of myself I hold in my brain, it will try to accomplish or make happen."

A place for you to reflect

My feelings:

My goals:

What I'm grateful for:

My progress:

Reminder:

Mental exercise:

Chapter Twenty-Seven:

Overcoming

I have always considered myself an overcomer, but when I had a stroke I became *the* overcomer. I had to. I had to overcome distance and learn to walk again. I had to overcome time and learn to wait. I had to overcome depression and be more positive. I had to overcome steps and new obstacles and pain and frustration and wanting results *now*. Overcoming became my new best friend. To overcome is hard work and it makes me tired. Naps are great.

The list of things to overcome is different for each person. But to overcome is a necessity. It is also a very honorable thing to do. Yet, when I am in the middle of a struggle to overcome something, I don't think of honor, I think of necessity. It is what I need to do at that moment in time. Later I can reflect on how far I have come and on what I have struggled to accomplish. Then I can appreciate the honor and progress.

I suggest no particular religion, but as each person walks his or her own spiritual path, the overcoming is the challenge. The Bible, near the end, in Revelations 21:7, says, "He that overcomes shall inherit all things." This particular path of overcoming is not what I would choose, but I am here on this particular path. Overcoming is a necessity. I am not waxing eloquent; I am just getting through the day and overcoming what I need to.

Some things are easier than others to overcome. Some tasks require more effort than others. Sometimes I have more physical pain than other times. Sometimes I have to ask for help. I don't know about other people, but with me, asking for help is difficult in its own right and has its own set of "overcoming" challenges.

With time, overcoming pays off, and some tasks get easier. The difficulty for many of us is in the waiting; overcoming the slow process of healing requires great patience.

There were times when there was darkness all around, and I could see the crevices of depression everywhere. It was at these times, when I was surrounded by doubt and fear, that I held on to my faith in a good God. I felt the winds of his love and grace fill my sails and lift me out of the darkness. I found it deep inside myself. I suggest that you do it as well. It is different for each person. But it is there, nonetheless. Look for his grace, and it will greet you lovingly every time. Overcoming will become a way of life. As you struggle and win, the frustration will ease, and you will become an overcomer.

Daily practices

Feelings: I feel that I am turning some invisible corner of healing. I am the same as yesterday, but I am hopeful.

Goals: My goal is to continue to heal.

What I'm grateful for: I am grateful for small amounts of progress and for large amounts.

Progress: My progress is made in small ways, but the small progress adds up. I am worlds ahead of where I was.

Reminder: I tell myself, "Whatever I need to do today, God will help me do it. I need also to remember that my efforts are incredibly important—and I need to hold in my mind the image of me completely well."

Mental exercise: I affirm, "The brain is a magnificent organ; whatever image of myself I hold in my brain, it will try to accomplish or make happen."

A place for you to reflect

My feelings:

My goals:

What I'm grateful for:

My progress:

Reminder:

Mental exercise:

Chapter Twenty-Eight:

Transforming

Transforming is what the caterpillar does when it becomes a butterfly. It spins a cocoon and waits, and one day it becomes a butterfly. It sounds easy: 1–2–3. But it is not that easy. I don't know what triggers each step of the process. I know that when it is time for the butterfly to emerge, the coming out of the cocoon is very difficult for the butterfly. It struggles and struggles and struggles. It almost dies in the process.

When I had a stroke, it happened in an instant. I didn't think of it at the time, but I was instantly wrapped in a cocoon. From that moment on, recovery was to become my new focus. I didn't think about that either. I had to be taught how to recover.

For months I struggled to get out of my own personal cocoon. As I struggled, I believed that I would be getting back to the way I was before the stroke. But in all honesty, I think I am becoming a new creature, like the butterfly. I am not getting back to "normal." I am becoming something else. I don't think I will ever be the same again. I don't think I will be less than I was. I think I will be more than I was. Like the caterpillar, I will crawl and struggle until I am transformed and can fly like the butterfly.

It is part of this transformation to think of myself as more, not less. The butterfly is changed physically. I am changed physically and mentally and spiritually. I am beginning to see myself differently in my mind. I know that I am more. There are times I feel that I am less because of the stroke, but then I realize that I am actually more. "Less is more," in a strange way.

Let me say very emphatically that the change has taken time and patience, and a lot of both, for me. This butterfly is becoming a new creature slowly. The operative descriptions above are: *becoming, new creature*, and *slowly*. Much of the time the operative word is *slowly*. I am impatient, and I want it now. For me, part of becoming a new creature is becoming more patient. In time I will be transformed.

It is anybody's guess what or whom I will become, but it is my best guess that the "new me" will be a more positive, stronger, and improved creature.

One of the most beautiful and mystical quotes from the Bible is from the book of Isaiah, in chapter 43, verse 19. God said to Isaiah, "Behold, I will do a new thing; now it shall spring forth; shall you not know it? I will even make a way in the wilderness and rivers in the desert." I love this thought. God is doing a new thing in me. Awesome. If he is doing something new, it is most probably a good thing. It is a very good thing. My advice to you is to let him do that new thing in you.

Life is change for all of us, every day, so let that change be good. Be the new creature. Be transformed into that beautiful person you are becoming.

Daily practices

Feelings: I feel partly transformed, but I am going in the right direction.

Goals: My goal is to heal.

What I'm grateful for: I am grateful when I heal in small ways. It is working.

Progress: I am making progress day by day.

Reminder: I tell myself, "Whatever I need to do today, God will help me do it. I need also to remember that my efforts are incredibly important—and I need to hold in my mind the image of me completely well."

Mental exercise: I affirm, "The brain is a magnificent organ; whatever image of myself I hold in my brain, it will try to accomplish or make happen."

A place for you to reflect

My feelings:

My goals:

What I'm grateful for:

My progress:

Reminder:

Mental exercise:

Chapter Twenty-Nine:

Envisioning

The process of envisioning is perhaps the most mystical of all. The brain is so powerful that what it sees, or envisions, it will bring to pass in our lives. If I hold thoughts of failure in my brain as a vision for my future, it will find a way to make failure the reality. If I hold thoughts of success for myself in my brain, it will make success the reality. It sounds easy, and it is easy. The challenge is to imagine only positive visions. I need to see myself overcoming all obstacles and achieving my goals. This was easy for me to say before—when I was the person that had not had a stroke. But I did have a stroke. So now I need to see myself as being completely well.

I need to envision new neural pathways opening in my brain to allow my body to do all it needs to do with my leg, my foot, my arm, my hand, and my voice.

Sometimes my leg or arm shakes back and forth. Physical therapists call it *clonus*. I found I could stop the shaking by putting weight or pressure on the limb. Now I've come to realize that I can stop it another way—with my mind! I think the words "stop it," and it stops! It is hard to believe, but I have found that it works. Sometimes it works better than other times. Sometimes I have to be persistent. But it works. The brain is powerful. The brain will work for me with my own body. It will also work for me to bring about what I need to happen in my life. This concept goes into another zone. This is a little much for some folks. But I know it is true. I have known it for years. I have never had a need to put it to work like I do now.

You may be thinking that this won't work, but how do you know it won't work? I can't prove that it will work, but you can't prove that it won't work either.

So give it a chance, okay? Try it! You have time to try this new idea out. Practice it. Take this practice out for a spin. Hold the idea in your head that you are getting better, and you will get better. What do you have to lose? It worked for me. It may work for you. What if it makes you better? Let this thought sink in: *What if it makes me better?*

I am practical person. I do what works. I am not a theorist; I am a pragmatist. I can assure you, this works.

The bottom line is this: see it in your mind consistently and persistently, and it will come to pass, if that is what God has planned for you. Sounds simple? Sounds a little like hocus-pocus? Hold the vision in your mind and you can make it come true.

Envisioning the positive changes that you want in your life is not a new concept. Many people may think that it is, but it has worked for centuries. A quote from chapter 23, verse 7 in the book of Proverbs, in the Old Testament, says, "As he thinks in his heart, so is he." This is the same thing put a little differently. Put this powerful practice to work in your life.

Daily practices

Feelings: I feel I have a part in my own healing.

Goals: My goals are to do my part and envision my progress, and to do my physical therapy.

What I'm grateful for: I am grateful for the progress I am making; it is sure and steady.

Progress: I am making progress each day.

Reminder: I tell myself, "Whatever I need to do today, God will help me do it. I need also to remember that my efforts are incredibly important—and I need to hold in my mind the image of me completely well."

Mental exercise: I affirm, "The brain is a magnificent organ; whatever image of myself I hold in my brain, it will try to accomplish or make happen."

A place for you to reflect

My feelings:

My goals:

What I'm grateful for:

My progress:

Reminder:

Mental exercise:

Chapter Thirty:

What I Have Learned

This chapter is developing over time, but I can describe what has happened so far with my attitude and outlook.

1. I found that I had to be more patient with myself.
    I had to be kind to myself and love myself. What I had done quickly before the stroke, now took more time and patience. I had to be more methodical and more deliberate. I had to slow down the speed of getting things done and increase the effort it took to accomplish the task. I was a different person now. My life had changed. When I had the stroke—that moment—I felt that my life became undefined, and now it was up to me to redefine it.

2. After the stroke I realized how immediate life is.
    It put me in the "now" more of the time. I am in touch, in a more real way, with how temporary and how impermanent life can be. I only have so much time. And I have none to waste on the things that don't matter, at least to me. This is my life, and I am accountable for it and for its accomplishments. If this sounds selfish, well, it is. It is up to me to make the most of this life and the time I have with this earthly existence. No one will do it for me. People will help me if I ask them, but I need to ask. I alone am responsible for doing it, whatever "it" is. I knew this before; now it seems to be more real somehow.

3. After the stroke I found that I was less tolerant of that which is insincere.
    I became less patient with what is not authentic. I had no time left for those things and those people who wasted my time.

4. I have learned to measure success in different ways.

    Before, I believed success meant getting things accomplished. Since simple tasks can be difficult for me now, I measure success differently. Everyday tasks can mean success for me now: climbing the stairs, using the toilet, taking a shower, cooking my own breakfast, washing my dishes, or doing my laundry. Folding my clothes is something to watch, I suspect. I get the job done, but some might say it is difficult to watch. But I feel good about myself when I am finished. My high point came one week when, after working hard at the task, I was able to touch all the fingers on my left hand with my left thumb. It sounds easy, but it has taken a long time to accomplish. I take nothing for granted.

5. Acceptance is another thing that I learned.

    There were many low points, such as not making it to the bathroom in time, and being embarrassed and frustrated with myself. Now I listen more closely to my body, and I accept that I move more slowly than I used to.

6. I've learned I can never quit trying and that eventually persistence will cause my situation to improve.

7. I've also learned to keep my sense of humor close at hand.

8. During my darkest hours, my guardian angels were the closest.

    They encouraged me and made me want to try. I did my part; God did his. I am recovering.

9. Hope is extremely important. It is the life breath of the human spirit.

10. Overcoming the obstacles I face each day is my work each day.

11. I am being transformed in this situation to a life that is more, not less.

12. Envisioning my healing and holding a vision of my well self in my mind each day will advance me in that direction as quickly as possible.

Daily practices

Feelings: I have learned that feelings are important, but they are only feelings. I am healing each day.

Goals: My goal is to heal completely.

What I'm grateful for: I am grateful for all that does not need healing. I am grateful for all that I have. I have learned that my gratitude is a tool I use daily. It is a key to my healing. I am grateful for what I have, and God gives me more.

Progress: I climbed the stepladder and changed the lightbulbs in the garage-door opener. It was hard for me but I did it, and I didn't fall off the ladder. Pushing the limits of my stroke recovery helps me progress.

Reminder: I tell myself, "Whatever I need to do today, God will help me do it. I need also to remember that my efforts are incredibly important—and I need to hold in my mind the image of me completely well."

Mental exercise: I affirm, "The brain is a magnificent organ; whatever image of myself I hold in my brain, it will try to accomplish or make happen."

A place for you to reflect

My feelings:

My goals:

What I'm grateful for:

My progress:

Reminder:

Mental exercise:

The End

About the Author

Paul Sybert holds a bachelor of science degree in electrical engineering. He has worked as an engineer, a software analyst and programmer, a songwriter, and a minister. He has played his guitar and sung his songs in churches and coffee-houses. He is recovering from a stroke and currently lives in Endicott, New York.

978-0-595-46079-3
0-595-46079-8